Christina Czeschik

Ratko Stambolija

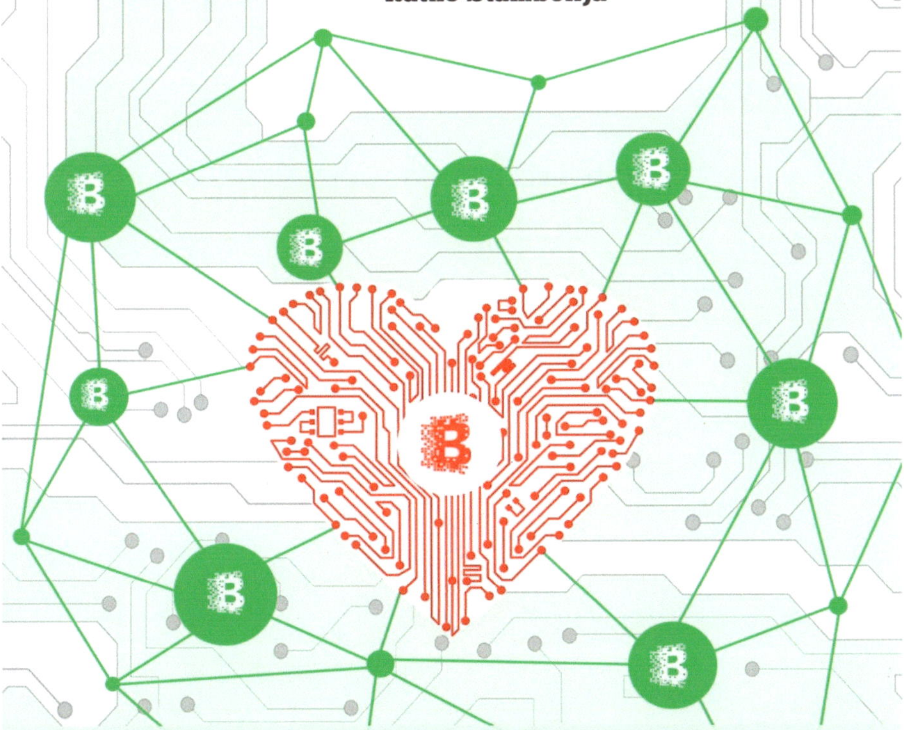

A Quick Guide to Blockchain in Healthcare

INTELLICORE PRESS

A Quick Guide to Blockchain in Healthcare

Christina Czeschik & Ratko Stambolija

Intellicore Press

March 2018

ISBN: 978-3-96214-005-2

Publisher:
Intellicore UG (haftungsbeschränkt)
Herkulesstr. 3-7
45127 Essen
Germany

Cover design by Nikola Borojević
Proofreading by Audrey Malone

Introduction

What is Blockchain, and how is it relevant to the healthcare industry?

This guide will answer both questions as well as demonstrate some practical uses and pilot projects of Blockchain in healthcare.

We will explain the technology in a clear and not-overly-technical manner, helping you – whether you are a physician, nurse, hospital administrator or technical staff – to understand future implications of Blockchain for your line of work and whether it has the potential to improve patient care. To achieve this, we will attempt to give a balanced account of both Blockchain's advantages as well as its potential pitfalls.

If you find this publication helpful, we kindly ask that you leave a review on Amazon.com or the online book retailer of your choice. But even more importantly, if you are missing something that we should cover here, if you find passages to be less than clear, or if you have any other suggestions for improvement, please do not hesitate to drop us an e-mail at blockchain@intellicore.press. We are looking forward to hearing from you!

Christina Czeschik and Ratko Stambolija

blockchain@intellicore.press

https://intellicore.press

And one last note before you dive into our little book: We provide assistance and consulting services for **Blockchain projects**, specifically **whitepaper** concepts, writing and editing services, as well as **PR services**, in a variety of industries.

To learn more, visit us at: https://www.intellicore.press

Contents

Digitalization of Healthcare

In an increasingly interconnected world, in which users have come to expect a fast and consistent stream of information, new technologies are often embraced by society and industries almost as soon as they become available. However, the healthcare industry is falling behind in the adoption of new technologies, despite all available innovations and economical requirements.

Many key institutions acknowledge that stakeholders in the healthcare industry should play active roles in forming new infrastructures for the industry and its users, regardless of who they may be — government agencies, drug developers, hospitals administrators, nurses, doctors or patients.

The future of healthcare IT lies in interoperability, achieved by creating open formats and standards that can be widely adopted and exchanged in the industry. Interoperability is important for the implementation of electronic health records (EHR), making the exchange of health-related information between involved parties more efficient. Safe storage of all information gathered by healthcare agents with the highest regard to privacy of patients is important as well.

In this book, we explain the potential healthcare use of Blockchain technology, a promising new framework for distribution and integration of healthcare data across a range of different uses. It offers a solution for several issues with existing, centralized systems and allows the creation of more efficient, decentralized and secure systems. We will also list some examples of companies that have already implemented Blockchain systems or are working on implementation in the healthcare field.

In the end, we hope that you'll close this book feeling well equipped to make an informed decision about whether or not a blockchain-based solution is right for your institution or practice.

What is Blockchain, and How Does It Work?

Blockchain technology was presented in a 2008 paper by Satoshi Nakamoto (a pseudonym for an unknown person or group of persons) as a decentralized, cryptographically empowered currency framework for financial transactions without an intermediary. Digital currency is not a completely new idea; however, Nakamoto's paper offered a solution for the "double spending" problem: How do you prevent a person from replicating their digital currency and spending it multiple times? Blockchain was a solution to this problem that led to the establishment of the most popular digital currency to date: Bitcoin.

So, what is the Blockchain?

Fundamentally, the Blockchain is a shared database but with one key difference. As opposed to a traditional (e.g., relational) database, there is no central ownership. Instead, information is managed through the consensus of network members who work together (with the assistance of cryptography) to choose what is included in the database — in the Blockchain. Every member keeps an identical, full copy of all transactions ever made in the network to ensure that no duplicate transactions are entered into the database. The network can be public (like Bitcoin, open to anybody) or private (allowed only for certain individuals).

When new data needs to be added, every machine on the network is notified and updates its copy of the Blockchain accordingly. The outcome is a far-reaching and decentralized source of trust — formed through cryptographically aided consensus. The stored data can be anything: financial transaction, personal identity, land titles, intellectual property, even "smart contracts" — special computer code executed when certain pre-defined conditions are met. Still, Blockchain's most important trait is its immutability: once something has been placed on the Blockchain, it becomes permanent — spread across many computers, cryptographically secured and added to the history of transactions.

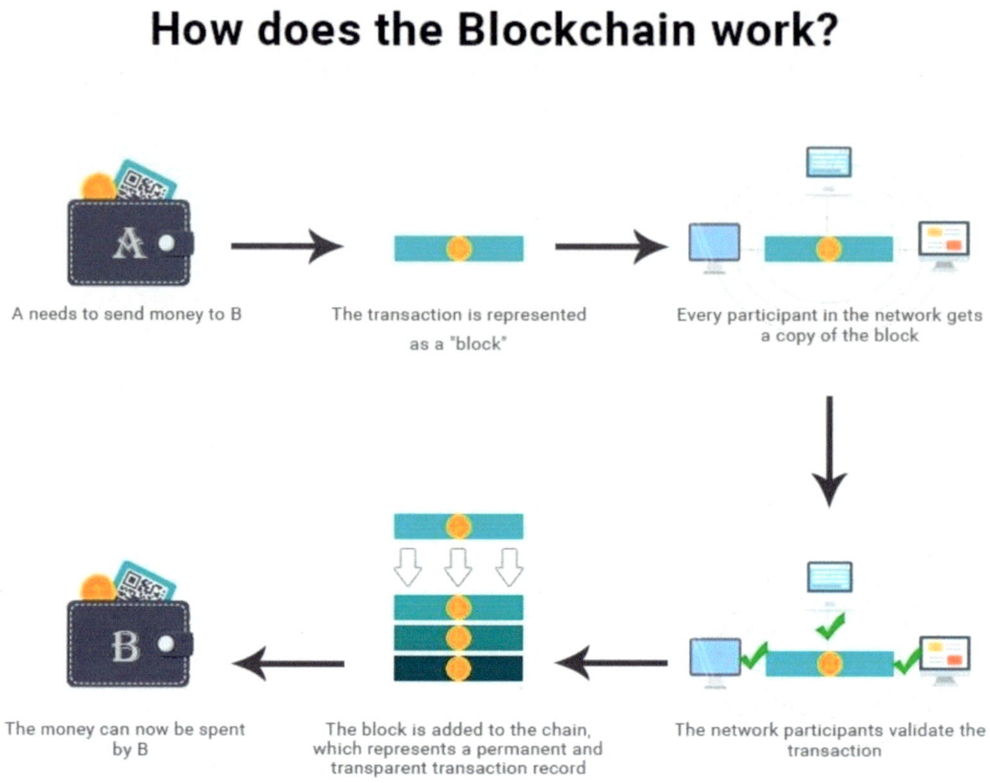

Figure 1. The principle behind Blockchain, illustrated with a Bitcoin transaction.

Thus, the Blockchain is often compared to a ledger. As in a traditional paper-based ledger, you can only append data and can never delete or manipulate existing data. The crucial distinction between the two is, of course, that the Blockchain is present in many identical copies on many different computers.

Bitcoin was the first project powered by a Blockchain. It was followed by numerous other so-called cryptocurrencies — Litecoin, Dogecoin, Ether, ZCash, just to name a few. Cryptocurrencies are called "crypto" not because transactions are anonymous. In fact, transactions in most cryptocurrencies are merely pseudonymous, meaning that for all transactions, they are transparent for all participants' addresses (pseudonyms) involved. True, if you change addresses frequently enough, you can achieve anonymity, and there are several currencies now – ZCash, PIVX, and others – that have been designed for real anonymity using advanced mathematical concepts of zero-knowledge proofs. However, anonymity is generally not a feature of cryptocurrencies and not of Blockchains employed for other purposes than cryptocurrencies.

Rather, cryptocurrencies were named this way because cryptography plays an important role in how permissions to spend currency units are managed. We will explain this in greater detail in the following section, but the gist of it is: The person who creates a transaction — who "spends" currency units — signs this transaction with a private key. Roughly, this corresponds with the physical signature on a check. Each private key has a corresponding public key that is available to the public. Everyone with access to this public key can check the integrity of the signature that was performed using the corresponding private key, making it even more secure against forging than a traditional pen-on-paper signature (provided everyone is keeping their private keys safe).

For what other purposes besides cryptocurrencies is the Blockchain used? As we will see below, one of the major advantages of the Blockchain is the potential to make a central trusted authority for transactions redundant. Transactions here are defined as the transfer of a right, for example, the right to spend a certain amount of currency. Thus, while financial institutions first viewed Blockchain as a freakish hype that would soon fade, and later as a potential threat to their business models, many are now developing models of how to make the Blockchain work for them, to carry out transactions between participants that do not necessarily trust each other, in a resource-efficient manner. Similarly, Blockchains can be employed to manage property other than money, for example, instead of a traditional land registry. However, the Blockchain cannot only help to manage property rights, it may be useful as well to manage access rights to one's medical records, as we will see below. But first, some technical terms.

Technical Blockchain Terms Explained

The three main components of a Blockchain are:

- A network of computers,
- a network protocol, and
- a consensus mechanism.

Various Blockchain configurations use different consensus mechanisms, depending on the type and size of the network and the goal of a specific group or company. The Bitcoin Blockchain, for example, is public and **permissionless**, which means that anyone can participate and add blocks to the ledger — provided they have sufficient computation power, as we will explain below. As an alternative, many companies are exploring private or **permissioned** Blockchains whose networks consist only of known (invited) participants. Most healthcare Blockchain projects are based on permissioned Blockchains.

Everyone with a networked computer may participate in a (permissionless) Blockchain's network. Each computer in a specific network is called a node. If everything is running per protocol, each node should have a copy of the entire ledger, which is sort of a local database, and should work with other nodes to keep the ledger's consistency intact. This creates **fault tolerance**, so if one node disconnects or goes down, no data is lost.

Whoever creates a **transaction** signs this transaction with a **private key**. Each private key has a corresponding **public key** that can be made available to everyone without compromising security. On the contrary, public availability of the public key is necessary to allow every network participant to check the integrity of the transaction. Private keys, however, must be guarded carefully by their owners, since ownership in a Blockchain system (be it of cryptocurrency units or other digital assets like reading permissions to a patient file) entirely depends on who is controlling the private key to a transaction. The underlying principle is that of public key cryptography, also used in other domains such as e-mail encryption (PGP, S/MIME) and digital signatures.

The **consensus mechanism** is a set of rules utilized by the network to verify each transaction and confirm the current state of the Blockchain. With Bitcoin as well as in the Ethereum Blockchain, on which currently most industry projects are based, the consensus mechanism is called **proof of work**, in which the network's participants run algorithms to confirm the digital signatures attached to blocks and verify each transaction.

After a transaction is executed on a node, the result becomes a proposed modification of the Blockchain's data. Other nodes in the network, which work on creating blocks out of single transactions, check whether the transaction is **valid**. A valid transaction does not contradict transactions in previous blocks or transactions that are candidates for inclusion in the same, current block. Approved transactions are placed into a block and re-distributed to all nodes in the network, which verify it again to ensure their records match. Typical transactions can be executed in milliseconds.

In blockchain networks that employ proof of work as the consensus mechanism, every time a network participant wants to create a new block out of several current transactions, it is necessary to solve mathematical problems that are artificially made difficult and computationally expensive. The purpose of this – the proof of work – is to keep malicious network participants from falsifying the current state of the Blockchain, to fool other participants into thinking, for example, that they have received digital currency while in fact the malicious participant has sent the currency units to an own account. The effort that goes into performing proof of work for the creation of new blocks is known as **mining**, and the participants or their computers performing this work are called **miners**. In Bitcoin, they are rewarded with digital currency; in other Blockchains, for instance in healthcare, that have no native currency, new concepts for rewarding miners need to be designed to keep the Blockchain mechanism intact.

The probably most popular alternative to proof of work right now is **proof of stake**. Here, in order to avoid malicious interference with the blockchain consensus, the creators of new blocks don't need to prove that they have invested time and energy to solve artificial mathematical problems, as in proof of work. Rather, they need to prove that they hold a certain amount of the underlying currency – that they have a "stake" in this currency. In most systems with proof of stake, the likelihood for each participant to be allowed to create the next block depends on the amount of currency they have staked. Sometimes, other factors come into play, such as the age of the staked coins, and/or a bit of randomness.

Critics say that proof of stake contradicts the original idea of cryptocurrencies – that is, to create a decentralized system. Power in these networks is concentrated with those who own lots of currency (any similarity to real-world systems being purely coincidental here, of course). However, proof of work is not an optimal solution for decentralized systems either, as experiences with Bitcoin have shown. Because of scaling effects, mining power in proof of work networks tends to centralize in the hands of the few as well.

It is probably safe to say that the search for a truly decentralized and equal consensus mechanism is still going on.

Advantages of Blockchain

Consensus without Trusted Intermediary

The Blockchain can create what is commonly called "consensus without trust". That is, the consensus mechanism as described above ensures a consensus throughout the network about the current state of the Blockchain—which transactions and blocks are valid, and which are not.

This is the responsibility of a central, trusted intermediary in a traditional system. In the case of financial transactions between individuals, this intermediary might be a bank. In the case of real estate transactions, it is the land registry. In healthcare, it might be an individual's general practitioner or the hospital responsible for an inpatient treatment.

Trusted intermediaries do not only require effort to establish them and considerable funds to run them. They also almost always come with certain questions, which is the elephant in the room: Is the central authority trustworthy? Or, does it have its own hidden agenda and economic or political motives? Or, is it underfunded and thus negligent and unreliable?

The more parties with divergent interests are involved in transactions, the more difficult it is to reach consensus about what exactly is a trusted intermediary. Looking at healthcare systems, who is trusted by all to manage a central electronic patient record? In Germany, for instance, stakeholders' economic motivations in the ambulatory and stationary sectors are distinctly different. It seems unlikely that physicians in ambulatory medical practices would willingly give up control over their patient records in favor of the local hospital, or vice versa, and both are unlikely to relinquish control to the patients (admittedly, this is difficult for legal reasons as well).

With Blockchain, a central intermediary can be rendered unnecessary under specific circumstances. In other circumstances, the power of intermediaries can be limited to the management of partial databases, as we will see below.

Robustness

In Blockchain, data is stored redundantly on all servers of the P2P network. All servers have identical copies of the Blockchain. Thus, if one of the nodes ceases to function, if a server goes down, data can be recovered easily from any of the other nodes.

This fault tolerance or robustness is one of the characteristics that contributed to the Internet's success as well; it is a common feature in decentralized systems, i.e., systems that do not depend on a central server or a hierarchical structure. However, in the case of the Internet, data on one server may very well be lost if the server malfunctions. The Internet's robustness is instead a robustness of data transmission; if one or even several servers malfunction (i.e., cannot transmit data packages anymore), then packages will be re-routed via alternative ways. (With increasing capacities and decreasing data storage prices, however, the Internet moves in the direction of data redundancy as well. Many download servers, for example, have so-called mirrors that host the same content, and some servers are even dedicated to storing snapshots of the contents of all sites on the Web, such as the Wayback Machine.)

Regarding the Blockchain, this robustness means that malevolent attacks with the purpose of bringing down the system need to target each server in the network to be successful. In systems that depend on a central server, targeting the (though usually well-protected) central server can be enough to put a whole system out of service.

However, the data redundancy of the Blockchain leads us to its first disadvantage.

Disadvantages of Blockchain

Performance

The more redundant your data is, the better? No – there is a trade-off between redundancy and performance. In any system, if you spend all your time and computing power doing backups, productivity will plummet, and having the same data repeatedly is just not a very efficient way of using storage space.

In case of the Blockchain, there are two additional complications:

- If you store real-world data in the Blockchain, the Blockchain will get very large, very fast. Bitcoin, the oldest Blockchain, has a size of 160 GB as of March 2018. And in the case of Bitcoin, there is not much data in each transaction. If you were to save patient medication files on the Blockchain, for example, this size would be reached much more quickly and expand further. If you multiply this with the number of Blockchain network participants, which may be in the thousands or even millions, you have an enormous waste of storage space.

- If you work with smart contracts, each contract needs to be executed on every server of the Blockchain network. Thus, not only storage space is wasted but computing power (i.e., energy) as well. And, maybe more importantly, if the smart contract accesses an external database, every Blockchain server will access this database. For example, a smart contract for prescription management might want to access an external database of medication interactions. Apart from creating a lot of traffic, this comes with the risk that not every server will get the same data upon its request – maybe the medication interaction data are being updated while the Blockchain server is accessing it. This destroys the Blockchain consensus and thus its underlying principle.

There are a couple of approaches to solving the first problem. For example, storing only references and permissions on the Blockchain and not actual data will keep the Blockchain from growing quickly to a size that is no longer manageable. The actual data can be stored in external databases instead. For each record in an external database, a hash is calculated and stored in the Blockchain. The hash is a kind of checksum that will change every time the record changes the slightest bit. Thus, if the hash is saved in an immutable Blockchain block, one can check whether the record has been changed illegally by computing its hash and comparing it to the Blockchain content.

To address the second problem, the implementation of "oracles" has been suggested. These are external services that push necessary information into the Blockchain, instead of having the Blockchain servers pull the information from outside sources. Smart contracts should then only be used as a last resort, if the computational logic cannot be implemented any other way.

Privacy

The story of Blockchain and privacy is a story full of misunderstandings, one might say. The public tends to think of Bitcoin as an anonymous currency, allowing drug and weapon dealers on the darknet to conduct their business in complete obscurity. This is not so.

Instead, Bitcoin and other Blockchains are inherently transparent. They need to be because each node must be able to check the validity of transactions. The Blockchain is, however, in most cases pseudonymous. This means that the participants' personal identification is not stored directly on the Blockchain. In Bitcoin, for example, everyone can see which public keys are involved in a transaction. Each public key corresponds to an individual person or entity. Thus, if you observe the network long enough, you can derive some conclusions about who is who. Similarly, if you were to observe the transactions on an individual's traditional bank account, without knowing the name of this individual, after some time you would have a good idea to whom this account might belong.

Those who use Bitcoin for illegal purposes know that this makes them vulnerable to law enforcement and take countermeasures. They switch key pairs frequently, so that each public key is only used for one single transaction and then discarded.

In the context of healthcare, who performs transactions with whom can be privacy-sensitive. For example, a patient might not want his general practitioner (GP) to know that he has consulted a specialist for venereal diseases, even if the GP cannot see what exactly has been discussed in this consultation.

To preserve privacy in the Blockchain, one can adopt the approach taken by darknet dealers and switch public keys or pseudonyms frequently. Another approach is currently being developed that allows for real anonymity on the Blockchain, using the mathematical device of zero-knowledge proofs, as implemented in ZCash, for example.

How Can the Blockchain be Applied to Healthcare?

Knowing the advantages and pitfalls of the Blockchain raises the question: What can the Blockchain do for healthcare?

The applications of Blockchain in healthcare can be divided into five distinct fields:

- Electronic health record (EHR) management
- Medication planning and management
- Revenue cycle
- Logistics and supply chain in healthcare
- Connected medical devices

Electronic Health Record (EHR) Management

Most healthcare systems around the world suffer from data siloing and a lack of interoperability between domains. Current healthcare record systems – in the US, for example, as well as in Germany – are composed of an enormous number of disconnected databases. Medical history is divided and siloed, keeping doctors and patients from building complete health records. Records are usually spread across various institutions and suppliers that often use incompatible databases. Many hospitals, pharmacies and other users in the industry still cannot share information easily and digitally, and often, the fallback is to have the patient carry a piece of paper, e.g., a written report, which will then be entered into another provider's digital system again. This lack of interoperability leads to inefficiencies and errors.

In an ideal world, there might be an integrated EHR in which all medical information pertaining to a patient are collected – and this EHR would be controlled by the patient. It would be accessible from any medical institution at any time, provided that the patient gives consent and permission.

In most countries, this is only a faraway vision appearing on the horizon – visible only in good weather. In Germany, for example, a fully functional electronic health card (elektronische Gesundheitskarte, eGK), containing among other things a cryptographic key to a fully functional telematics infrastructure for the healthcare system, was supposed to be introduced in 2006. Finally, the card was distributed in 2015, replacing the old monofunctional cards. As of today,

March 2018, patients and providers are still waiting for the first useful applications of the eGK, like, for example, an integrated EHR.

However, because the need for such an integrated EHR is widely recognized, there are a number of pilot projects: A consortium led by Aachen University Hospital has developed an electronic case file (elektronische Fallakte, EFA), and insurer TK together with IBM has presented an electronic health record (elektronische Gesundheitsakte, eGA). Furthermore, there are some players in the market who focus on easing data exchange between providers without implementing a full EHR. One such company is connectedhealth.eu, offering a simple solution for PDF-based data exchange using patients' smartphones, called LifeTime.

A good EHR is not only defined by its logistics. Any solution that wants to be viable in a healthcare context – especially in privacy-conscious Germany, but in other countries as well – needs to take the principles of privacy and security into serious consideration. In Germany, implementation of the telematics infrastructure has repeatedly been delayed and even stopped by the General Meeting of the Federal Chamber of Physicians (Deutscher Ärztetag). The Chamber had formed the opinion that the solution in its then present state was not compatible with principles of privacy and informational self-determination for both patients and physicians.

This was reflected in a new e-health law which became effective in 2016. Data privacy and security for patients was prioritized highly in this law. However, regarding the technological implementation, the law remained vague.

Looking at other countries, especially those that do not have statutory health insurance as Germany has, the issue of security against malicious attacks and tampering becomes even more pressing: In the US, healthcare fraud is a substantial problem. Per the FBI, healthcare fraud costs the US tens of billions of dollars each year. Only a small fraction of this amount is recovered with the help of the authorities. Also, breaches in the past have led to hundreds of thousands of patients' records being offered on the black market.

Thus, a system is needed that is both robust against outside attacks and able to offer patients full control over permissions to use their data.

Can Blockchain be a technology to build an EHR system upon that is both secure and privacy-friendly and empowering patients to govern their own data?

This question was answered with a clear "yes" by, for example, MIT Media Lab and collaborators who developed the project MedRec (more about this in the section MedRec). Administering health data on the Blockchain enables patients to take back control over their data without involving middle men and gatekeepers any more, giving and revoking permissions freely and without significant delay. The giving and revoking is protocolled in a transparent manner on the Blockchain. This is advantageous for the physician as well, since she can prove which information have been available to her at a certain point in time, and which have not.

The use of smart contracts furthermore enables efficient automatization of processes: For example, a patient might automatically receive a patient history questionnaire upon the commencement of a new physician-patient relationship. Or a patient might receive automatic reminders to consult the doctor for certain preventive measures once a certain diagnosis is documented on the Blockchain, for example ultrasound examinations in case of pregnancy or dental examinations prior to heart valve surgery. Mechanisms like this could be implemented in other infrastructures as well – but on the Blockchain, the fact whether or not these reminders and the corresponding examinations have taken place are documented in a tamper-proof way in the patient's history.

Further options for the improvement of quality of care and patient safety, as well as automatization of processes, can be realized with medication planning on the Blockchain, integrated into an EHR or as a standalone system.

Medication Reconciliation and Patient Safety

Medication reconciliation is certainly one of the most important tasks related to patient management. Even when the patients can precisely recall all of their medications, errors in prescription records are a common occurrence. A study published in the American Journal of Managed Care in 2015 found that 77 percent of patients have discovered disparities or mistakes in their active medication records, while another study found that nearly 60 percent of patients taking opioids are likewise taking other medicines that could result in serious injuries or deadly interactions.

Patient safety is not only a concern of quality of care. Incidents can bring about severe financial punishments for hospitals and other medical facilities that do not prevent avoidable harm to the patient.

While there are already a number of systems addressing the issue of medication management, this is a challenge in which the innate capabilities of the Blockchain can be demonstrated very well. For example, when a physician writes a prescription for a medicine that negatively interacts with medication prescribed by another doctor, a smart contract on the Blockchain could detect the interaction and reject the second prescription (see figure 2).

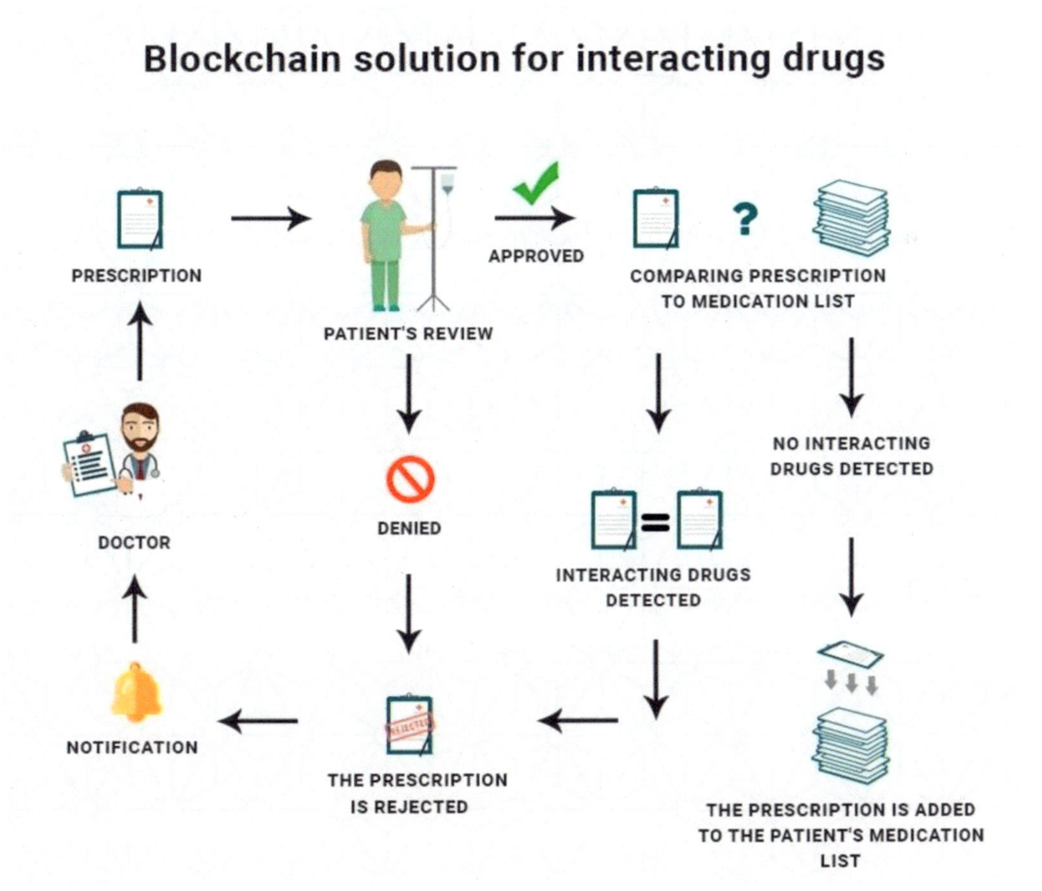

Figure 2. Managing prescriptions on the Blockchain.

If, however, there is no need for further discussion of the prescription, there is an automatic reconciliation of the new prescription with all other current medication on the Blockchain. This may for example be realized using a smart contract accessing an external database with medication interaction information (for disadvantages of accessing external databases, see section Performance). Alternatively, the interaction check might be part of the validation process as performed by the miners: They check whether there are relevant interactions before including the new transaction in a block.

In a similar manner, the ending a drug treatment can go through the same process, checking instead if there are any contraindications for stopping the treatment. The time interval during which a certain medication has been applied will remain on the Blockchain for the lifetime of the patient. Anonymized data from these sources can be used for research purposes as well.

Beyond the direct physician-patient relationship, when a care provider writes a prescription for a controlled substance, such as mood lifters, or a pharmacy fills that prescription, each pharmacy in the region could be easily informed about it, preventing abuse and fraud.

If a patient attempts to remove a pharmaceutical from the record on his or her own, a healthcare provider could receive a notice that may start a discussion about potential side effects as the reason for the removal of the pharmaceutical or the need to make improvements to the care plan.

However, these functions need to be balanced with patient autonomy over data. Can the patient manually prevent the pharmacy from knowing about previously filled prescriptions for potentially addictive substances? There is a spectrum of attitudes that range from old-fashioned medical paternalism (the doctor knows best) to giving the patient complete freedom to harm himself. Society needs to find the optimum of patient autonomy as a compromise between those two extremes.

Revenue Cycle

The Blockchain, especially in combination with smart contracts, has considerable potential for rendering the revenue cycle more tamper-proof and – by automating processes – more efficient.

When information about diagnoses and procedures are stored on the Blockchain or in external databases, with the datasets' signatures being part of the Blockchain, there is little opportunity to manipulate these information in order to increase revenue. If sufficiently good text mining software is available, the whole revenue cycle might even be automated in such a way that manual data entry is not necessary beyond the direct documentation of patient findings and procedures in the EHR.

As a speculative vision, if cryptocurrencies – such as Bitcoin or Ether – become more mainstream in the future, even the payments themselves might be executed by smart contracts, based on information that is available completely in or from the Blockchain.

Logistics and Supply Chain in Healthcare

Healthcare, just like any other big industry, has its own supply chains that are managed in large parts in an analog manner or, if digitally, with poorly defined processes for data exchange.

An industry's logistics can profit from Blockchain technology especially if there is a high risk of counterfeited or substandard products entering the supply chain. In healthcare, this is no different. The most sensitive areas here are pharma and medical devices with their components. In the pharma field, the electronic ePedigree system has been implemented to enable surveillance of each individual package of a drug. In the ONC Blockchain Challenge of 2016 (described further in sections MedRec and Other Winners of ONC Blockchain Challenge), IBM submitted a paper in which they proposed a Blockchain-based addition to the regular ePedigree system.

In a Blockchain-based system, suppliers can more easily be held accountable for the quality of their products. When each supplier stores in- and outgoing deliveries on the Blockchain, signed with his private key, a smart contract can check whether the number of outgoing products is higher than the number of incoming certified parts would make plausible. The smart contracts might then alert the supplier and/or customer, and possibly the authorities. In transactions in which no conflicts are detected, even the payment might be automatized.

Connected Medical Devices

There is an Internet of Things (IoT) in healthcare now as well: Medical devices communicate with each other via WiFi, Bluetooth and other interfaces. This leads to new vulnerabilities, in which infusion pumps or implants can be manipulated by outsiders, as the media has repeatedly reported.

One possible way of securing the interactions of connected medical devices is a public key infrastructure (PKI). Each connected device receives a public-private key pair, just like a person that communicates via encrypted e-mail, for example. The device's identity and its public key are confirmed in a certificate. Devices can now sign messages with their private key and thus prove their identity and provenance to other devices in the network.

If each message is stored as a transaction on the Blockchain, the history of messages remains transparent and tamper-proof. When there is a critical incident compromising patient safety, the Blockchain can be audited to find out in a reliable way whether or not the incident was caused by technical malfunction, and further incidents can effectively be prevented.

Examples of the Blockchain Use in the Healthcare Industry

Most Blockchain-based systems in healthcare are only just in the pilot phase. This may change soon, and we hope to reflect this in future editions of this booklet.

There is quite significant uncertainty and fear of the unknown in the healthcare industry. In addition, healthcare professionals often operate under scarcity conditions – especially scarcity of time. Stakeholders in healthcare are usually unwilling to invest in risky projects. However, to get the field of Blockchain in healthcare started, the US government entity ONC (The Office of the National Coordinator for Health IT) announced a competition for white papers on Blockchain in healthcare in summer of 2016. We will outline some of the 15 winners here, as well as some other promising projects and organizations.

MedRec

MedRec is a healthcare record system based on the Ethereum protocol developed for organization and management of medical files. It was developed by MIT student graduates Ariel Ekblaw, Asaf Azaria, and Thiago Vieira, alongside with Senior Research Scientist Andrew Lippman and outlined in their paper A Case Study for Blockchain in Healthcare: "MedRec" prototype for electronic health records and medical research data. The system utilizes the Ethereum Blockchain to create a decentralized content management system for healthcare information across multiple providers.

The main objective of MedRec is to help patients retain control over their medical data. The way MedRec does this is by linking access to the patient's health records across the range of databases used by their doctors. By working as a link between siloed medical records kept in institutions, it can also add personal sources from popular applications such as Fitbit or 23andme.

Patient data is not stored on the Blockchain directly (for problems associated with direct storage of large datasets on the Blockchain, see section Performance), but rather in individual external databases. However, each external dataset is digitally signed, and the signature is stored in the Blockchain, thus proving that the external record has not been tampered with.

The problem of mining and how to reward miners in a system without a cryptocurrency is solved by MedRec in a novel way: Medical researchers function as miners for MedRec and are awarded access to census data of the health records. The data is anonymized, and thus patients' privacy is protected, and the collected data may be used for medical research by the miners. Essentially, this makes MedRec both a clinical Blockchain and a medical research Blockchain.

MedRec does not seem to have evolved beyond the pilot project stage yet; however, the startup SimplyVital Health (see below) is building upon MedRec foundations.

Other Winners of ONC Blockchain Challenge

Other participants of the Blockchain Challenge addressed other problems in healthcare besides EHR and medication management in their papers.

For example, a paper submitted by another MIT team outlined a concept for clinical studies in precision medicine, based on MIT's Blockchain technology OPAL/Enigma.

A special feature of OPAL/Enigma is the so-called multi-party computation (MPC) capability. In MPC, participants of a P2P network can compute a common result using individual datasets without the need for each participant to disclose her individual dataset to the others. Thus, MPC enables evaluation of research data without compromising individual patients' privacy and without requiring a central authority to handle these data. Furthermore, proprietary intellectual property of pharma companies and others can be used in the process – chemical structures of new drugs, for example – without the need to give up business secrets.

Other papers tackled the revenue cycle. For example, participant Kyle Culver proposed a concept in which hospitals can directly bill patients' health plans. For each patient case, clinical information are stored in an external database, which can be queried via an FHIR-compatible API. FHIR is a new standard for healthcare interoperability based on the well-established HL7 v2.

The National Quality Forum also proposed a concept involving FHIR: The Blockchain as a replacement for cloud-based data collection from patients' wearables. These data could then be used to improve recording and evaluation of patient-reported outcomes (PROM): Outcomes better suited to assess patients' wellness and capabilities under therapy than conventional clinical study outcomes. Data in the Blockchain would only be accessible with private keys of both patient and physician, preventing unauthorized access by others.

An overview of factors that currently impede the implementation of Blockchain in healthcare is given by participant Drew Ivan in his paper.

SimplyVital Health

The MedRec concept described above has served as the foundation for a new venture, SimplyVital Health, founded by Kat Kuzmeskas and advised by one of MedRec's co-authors, John D. Halamka, CIO of Beth Isreal Deaconness Medical Center and Harvard Medical School.

SimplyVital Health too focuses on EHR and patient data management on the Blockchain to improve information flow between different parties in the healthcare ecosystem. SimplyVital Health's executives stress that one of their main objectives is to enable value-based healthcare.

In contrast to many competitors (see below), SimplyVital Health does have a functioning clinical implementation, the ConnectingCare platform, which was piloted at the Hartford HealthCare Bone & Joint Institute of Hartford Hospital (Connecticut, USA) and in the iCare network.

While the MedRec concept included proof of work as a consensus mechanism, with physicians and researchers as miners, ConnectingCare has no such mining concept. Instead, it implements a more energy-efficient proof of stake mechanism.

To date, ConnectingCare offers an interface for physicians and other personnel. The patient interface, according to Kuzmeskas, is being developed in iterations designed to optimize usability. Ultimately, patients are supposed to access ConnectingCare through an interface that relieves them from the difficulties of private key management, similar to the user interface of cryptocurrency exchange Coinbase.

As of this writing, SimplyVital Health is preparing a token sale of its Health Cash (HLTH) token to fund the development of the Health Nexus, an open-source blockchain protocol for healthcare (also see chapter To ICO or Not to ICO? below).

PreScrypt

The REshape center, part of the Radboud University Nijmegen Medical Centre in the Netherlands, has designed a Blockchain proof of concept together with Deloitte and SNC Bank

N.V. The intended use case was to ease the process of getting repetitive treatment for patients with chronic health problems.

PreScrypt is intended to give patients with chronic health problems a current and complete overview of their treatment and a way to receive digital prescriptions. They may choose their pharmacy and the healthcare service provider with which to share their information. This minimizes loss of information and the uncertainty that some individuals who suffer from chronic illnesses face while obtaining repeat medications. This helps reduce the burden of disease in the long run. All participants can also confirm if the information is still valid, since the Blockchain registers all transactions. For example, medication suppliers can verify whether a certified doctor has signed the prescription and whether another person has used the same prescription to get medication.

PreScrypt also addresses the problem of how to link the physical identity of the healthcare service user to his or her digital identity on the Blockchain. In this cooperation, the SNC Bank provides the iDIN online identification service that PreScrypt uses for identification on the Blockchain. iDIN was originally created for identification in the banking sector, but can nowadays be used by Dutch citizens for other types of online identification as well.

Unfortunately, PreScrypt is not a complete project – the pilot project's website is down as of writing this. However, Deloitte has also taken part in the Blockchain Challenge described above with the white paper Blockchain: Opportunities for Health Care.

Gem Health

Gem is a US company that offers enterprise Blockchain services for various industries in the global market. They launched Gem Health as a network that supports the development of applications and sharing of infrastructure for the healthcare industry. Just as MedRec, the Gem Health Blockchain is also based on the Ethereum protocol. The first big healthcare company to partner with Gem Health Network is Philips, founding the Blockchain Lab as its development center.

The Gem Health Blockchain is embedded into GemOS, a system that also offers capabilities for data storage, smart contract applications, APIs, and identity management.

CEO and founder Micah Winkelspecht presented Gem's first healthcare application on the Consensus industry conference in May 2017. Gem's product is targeted towards health claims management and supposed to tackle the most pressing issues in this field: A lack of real-time transparency into claims transactions, and the slowness of payment processing as a problem that especially affects providers. Later, Gem announced their partnership with Scandinavian health-IT provider Tieto. Gem and Tieto will collaborate to build a blockchain that allows for better protection of patients' privacy and data autonomy in healthcare.

GuardTime and EHR in Estonia

Estonia, as the poster child of digitalization in healthcare and public management, has already digitized the healthcare records of one million citizens. In March 2016, the government announced a cooperation with Blockchain startup GuardTime to build a system for managing these EHR on a Blockchain – a project that has been concluded successfully in the meantime.

GuardTime has developed a special approach to security on the Blockchain: Its Keyless Signature Infrastructure (KSI) is an alternative to traditional public key infrastructures (PKI) that require public-private key pairs for authentication (also see section Technical Blockchain Terms Explained).

In January 2018, GuardTime announced a collaboration with the Government of Thailand to secure administrative documents on the KSI Blockchain. So far, EHR do not seem to be part of the project.

Hyperledger Healthcare

Hyperledger is an open source project hosted by The Linux Foundation with the aim to provide Blockchain technologies for various industries. Among Hyperledger's members, there are notable global players such as Intel, SAP, accenture, IBM, Daimler, Airbus and others. So far, Hyperledger has formed working groups for the industries Finance and Healthcare, and offers numerous informational and training resources on the Hyperledger website. Those interested in developing pilot projects for healthcare can join Hyperledger's Healthcare mailing list.

Several current healthcare startups in the blockchain space have based their software upon the Hyperledger framework: Medicalchain, Proof Work and Patientory.

Medicalchain

Like MedRec and SimplyVital Health, startup Medicalchain focuses on the efficient exchange on medical data in healthcare. The Medicalchain platform will run on an ERC-20-compatible token, the MedToken. A prototype has been presented in summer of 2017, the beta version launch is announced for spring of 2018.

MedToken will be used to incentivize and reward network participants who validate blocks, and will serve as a means of payment for value-added services such as teleconsultations. Patients may earn MedTokens by voluntarily granting access to selected parts of their medical data to pharma companies with marketing and research interests. Long-term plans include claims management in MedToken, too.

A pre-sale of MedTokens to selected investors and angel funds in January 2018 has resulted in $20 million USD for further development of the concept and technical solution. The ICO announcement is pending.

Medicalchain recently announced a partnership with London-based Groves Medical Group, preparing a pilot project due to start in July 2018.

Proof Work

A similar solution to Medicalchain was presented by Israel-based startup Proof Work and its founders Suter and Aharonovsky at Disrupt Conference in December 2017 in Berlin. In their "patient first" approach, data autonomy of the patient is paramount; however, like in Medicalchain, patients on the PROOF™ blockchain may decide to sell their health data to pharmaceutical companies.

In addition, developers of health apps and other medical IT solutions may provide patients with apps to manage analyze their health data on the blockchain, such as medication alarms, and ultimately to interface with wearables and other applications of the Internet of Things (IoT).

Proof Work are specifically describing their solution as HIPAA- and GDPR-compliant.

Patientory

While Patientory is also developing a framework for health information management on the Blockchain, their solution seems to be less focused on patient data autonomy and instead on social media features: A health-centered social network for patients.

Technically, Patientory's information management solution, self-described as HIPAA-compliant, builds upon an Ethereum-based data layer with an Oracle-based middleware that tackles management of smart contracts, identities and keys. Users will only interact with the upper presentation layer.

Patientory too uses a native currency on its platform, the PTOY. PTOY, according to Patientory, will be a means of payment "to rent health information storage space, and to execute health-specific smart contract payments and transactions".

PTOY have been sold to early investors in an ICO in summer of 2017. However, the ICO was received somewhat sceptically by the crypto community, apparently due to intransparencies and communication issues. However, the ICO has not been a fraud, as some very vocal adversaries have tried to predict; the company is still in place and, according to the website, working on the development of their solution.

To ICO or Not to ICO?

When reading about health blockchain startups, one concept that you may have noticed to pop up repeatedly is that of the Initial Coin Offering (ICO), also known as Token Generation Event (TGE), Token Sale or Crowdsale.

Originally, an ICO is exactly what the term suggests: Upon creation of a new cryptocurrency, the newly created coins are offered to the public for the first time, usually in exchange for other, established cryptocurrencies such as Bitcoin.

However, it didn't take long until blockchain startups noticed that an ICO for them was an interesting new way of raising venture capital. The idea is simple: Create a coin or "token" that integrates with the startup's software platform and sell this coin to the public in return for cryptocurrency or fiat currency (fiat meaning real-world currency such as US Dollar or Euro). This token does not need to be based on a blockchain that is self-developed from scratch – in fact, the most popular technological foundation for ICO tokens is the Ethereum blockchain, whose smart contracts offer a number of useful functionalities for blockchain platforms.

For a startup, an ICO has certain advantages over traditional venture capital: Because ICOs are accessible to small investors (in contrast to venture capital rounds), they do not only serve to raise capital, but they can also be an instrument in community building and user acquisition. Furthermore, they can be executed in a shorter timeframe and with less administrative and financial overhead than other ways to acquire funding.

What do investors get in return for their funds? This differs from startup to startup: Some tokens are so-called utility tokens that can be exchanged for goods and services on the platform. An example of this would be MedTokens, Medicalchain's platform currency. Other tokens are so-called equity tokens: They confer the right to vote, for example, to take profit shares, or to wield any other of the rights that come with traditional shares of stock. Where exactly the boundary between utility tokens and equity tokens lies, and which other kinds of tokens need to be distinguished, is a matter of ongoing debate between crypto investors and financial authorities. For the latter, this question is a salient one because it affects the legal status of tokens in most countries.

The problem with ICOs? Lack of regulation and the crypto investment bubble of 2017 have tempted many a crypto enthusiast to launch their own ICO for projects that were little more than an idea, or even outright fraud. When an ICO goes bad – i.e., when the funds are not used for purposes of development, as promised by the team, or when the team even vanishes completely, taking investors' funds with them – there is practically nothing the investor can do to about it.

Properly executed ICOs, on the other hand, even if they have less administrative and regulatory overhead than other ways of funding, do require a high effort in two domains: Legal counsel – and PR and marketing. The legal situation is constantly changing and varies significantly between countries, or even federal states within countries. PR and marketing are vital to reach a sufficiently large crowd – after all, this is crowdfunding.

So, is it a good idea to invest in the ICO of a healthcare blockchain startup? In most cases: No – it's wiser to wait and see if they are ever going to develop a working product. Among all ICOs, those with a demonstrably functional product are arguably the most likely to succeed, and may be considered by adventurous investors.

Benefits of Blockchain in Healthcare

Secure and Efficient Sharing of Data

Using a Blockchain enables hospitals, insurers, and laboratories to form real-time connections and share data instantly and consistently in a way that is secure and, to the patient, transparent. With the addition of smart contracts and similar constructs, there are many opportunities to render business processes more efficient by automatization, for example, by having smart contracts for provider payment depending on the services that a patient received.

Importantly, the Blockchain does not need to be implemented as the sole database system of a provider's organization, but can function as an auditable interface between standalone databases, improving efficiency and patient safety.

Medical research can profit from the opportunity to more easily perform longitudinal studies – something that is often hindered by incompleteness and siloing of centralized medical records and the inability to contact patients for their approval.

Encouraging the Work of Coordinated Healthcare Teams

In a similar vein, data management on the Blockchain will be useful for the implementation of so-called integrated healthcare models, in which the stationary and ambulatory sectors need to exchange information just in time to coordinate care and create an efficient and agreeable patient journey.

There is a substantial number of health-related information that has been gathered by healthcare providers and patients; however, it has not been converted to standard formats that empower an extensive individualized care plan that contributes to long-term patient health. This shows the key issue, as most the information is in individual data silos of a given institution and are not available for use by their system partners who are likewise engaged in patient care. If, on the other hand, the healthcare industry had individuals' records unified on a Blockchain-based care management platform, both providers and patients could cooperate in the joined effort of a healthcare team with individuals working at various facilities.

Patients would no longer oversee toting records back and forth between different institutions and appointments or precisely describing the therapy of one specialist when visiting another. Instead, providers can work together and communicate directly, while leaving the control of all edits and changes in the record in patients' hands.

Patients Keep Full Access and Control

In the Blockchain environment, users can keep full control of the information related directly to them, giving only access to the healthcare providers with which they want to share the data.

Instead of having one central database with an administrator that acts as a gatekeeper, there is a shared ledger spread across a network of synchronized, replicated databases, visible only to users who have access. As we have seen above, hacking one block of transactions in the chain is impossible without simultaneously hacking all other blocks in the chain's chronology. The patient's prescriptions, X-rays, blood analyses and other important medical data will be visible to the patient, and every change to these records would require the patient's approval.

In a Blockchain, as we have seen above, everyone in the participant group — patients, doctors or other providers — holds his own local duplicate of the shared dataset. When one entity wants to make a change or update that information, the potential edit must meet a number of cryptographic criteria that confirm the identity of a person or an entity looking to make the change. Everyone from the group must confirm the transaction to be valid before it can be verified. Then every locally stored copy of the information is changed per the activity performed.

The patient might define different sharing parameters for various types of information. For example, information about vaccinations can be viewed by any healthcare provider, information about blood type only by emergency health personnel, or information about mental health issues only by the mental health professional. Using an app or web portal, these permissions should be easily changeable by the patient.

The system could be set to send automated notifications when an entity asks for permission to access specific information or request to make a change to the record, giving people an additional layer of security and more control over how, when, and for what reason their information is shared.

Furthermore, as changes made to Blockchain all incorporate detailed timestamps, patients could possibly check all activity on their account from one place, preventing any possible confusion and setting higher accountability across the network. Having patients check their full records might lead to an increased workload for healthcare professionals first, needing to field questions by patients who are new to the form and language of healthcare records, but may prove to be an effective risk management tool later. Experience in healthcare shows that many errors in medication or other therapeutic issues are detected, not by healthcare professionals, but by patients and their families who were given access to this information. Arguably, no healthcare professional has as much time to spend on a single patient's record as the corresponding patient and family.

Improving the Patient Identification Process

Patients are not static creatures. They change names, move from one location to another, switch care providers, buy different insurance plans, have children, etc. Guaranteeing that a patient's identity is valid and current throughout his life journey along the care continuum without duplication, cancellation, or other errors is a very difficult task.

The greater part of health data management experts frequently experiences patient coordination issues, per a 2016 AHIMA report, and patient ID issues are at the top of industry lists of patient security risks and concerns.

Misidentification of patients could prompt administration of improper treatments due to the absence of vital healthcare information about the patient. This likewise creates a poor user experience for patients, who may ask why they need to tell their life stories all over again upon hospital admission, or who are unsettled when they discover that obsolete medication is still on their current records.

Thus, without a national patient identifier, Blockchain might be the next best thing for keeping people and their records together, creating a unified longitudinal healthcare record and tie information closely to the person.

Obviously, this would require something close to universal adoption of Blockchain technology and tools; however, medical institutions show genuine desire to make that happen, as seen in the following chapter.

Integrating the Healthcare Ecosystem

In summary, Blockchain technology offers many benefits to patients, healthcare service providers, medical researchers, and caregivers. The establishment of a single system to store all healthcare data, being able to track personal information in a real-time and enhancing security by putting in place permissions to access data at a granular level will serve both personalized medicine and medical research.

Healthcare researchers need access to comprehensive and broad sets of data to enhance the conceptualization of diseases, speed-up biomedical research, track drug development, design customized personal medication plans per the patient's genetics, environment, and lifecycle. Blockchain technology provides an environment that allows data sharing for these purposes. It can deliver a wide variety of data by encompassing patients from various social-economic and ethnic backgrounds and different geographical origins. The Blockchain offers access to the analytic data, which is perfect for longitudinal studies because it gathers healthcare data across the lifetime of the patient.

Using the technology in healthcare can allow the user to extend healthcare data acquisition to encompass those individuals who may be unable to take part in the research or those who are from currently underserved medical communities. The shared data platform can ease the process of contacting the difficult to reach portion of the population and hence generates highly relevant results to the overall public.

The data structures of the Blockchain technology will also be a great choice for collecting information from mobile applications and wearable sensors. The results will contribute much information on the benefits versus risks of medication alongside the reported outcomes from the patients. Additionally, using wearable sensors and mobile applications to combine health information with information from genomics and other fields will enhance medical researchers' capabilities, as they classify their patients into different categories, depending on how well they respond to treatment plans or those who are more vulnerable to specific diseases.

There is also a good chance that daily personalized health information will be used to improve patients' compliance and engage them in their healthcare. Additionally, the Blockchain may grant doctors the ability to obtain regular data for the patient, such as blood sugar levels or daily blood pressure readings, not only when the user goes in for a check-up. This process will, in turn, enhance individualized healthcare that will come with specialized medication plans while measuring treatment efficiency and outcomes.

Another advantage of the distributed system is that it would ensure continuous access and availability to real-time data as the best way to improve clinical care coordination and emergency care. Such data would also enable public health resources and researchers to quickly spot, isolate, and drive environmental condition changes that influence public health. For example, specialists would be able to detect epidemics by looking for an increase of infection cases in the day-to-day statistics. This would allow them to react early enough and contain them.

Availability of wearable sensor data and mobile applications in real-time would facilitate 24-7 monitoring of high-risk patients and support the invention of programs that would inform healthcare providers and caregivers whenever a patient reaches a critical state that requires action. The care teams would be able to reach out to their patients in time and plan for early intervention.

The healthcare Blockchain could be easily used to promote the development of healthcare programs. These applications would assist healthcare providers in searching for recent healthcare research and develop personalized medication plans. The patient and healthcare provider will get access to similar information and will be able to participate in educative and collaborative discussions regarding the best possible treatment choices not based on intuition and doctor experience but on actual research.

Possible Pitfalls of Blockchain in Healthcare

Of course, every technology has two sides – the Blockchain is no exception, as we have discussed above. Furthermore, there are some pitfalls of Blockchain that become relevant specifically when the Blockchain is used in a healthcare context.

User-controlled Data

Although it seems like a good idea to give users complete control of their medical records, there are also accompanying risks to this. The problem with giving patients' control can surface when the patient is incapacitated and the doctors at the emergency room need to gain access to medical records without the patient's permission. To prevent this lack of information about the patient when every second counts, a back door must exist. And this back door, in turn, is a security risk.

Besides that, with the use of private keys and wallets in the Blockchain system come additional risks and key management problems. The costs of training users on how to properly use their new healthcare system would be significant as well. And for those patients who are unable or unwilling to learn how the technology works, the likelihood of error rises, which could result in stolen or lost data. Other usability issues could also increase already high expenses of Blockchain implementation.

Vendor Lock-in

Vendors of permissioned Blockchains – the kind of Blockchain most prevalent in healthcare projects – are usually focused on keeping the customers locked into their platforms. By reaching out to the companies and attracting more users, they increase switching costs. This allows vendors to control user data and gives them the freedom to raise prices at will.

Companies working with Blockchain platforms know that once an application is built with their software, the costs of moving to another platform becomes prohibitively high. It may be a good idea to wait for established software vendors to support the integration of a new technology than to start building something from scratch.

Immature Infrastructures

Healthcare technology advances slowly – at least in the field, not necessarily in companies' labs. Reasons for this include high investments that have been made in legacy systems and the time-sensitive nature of day-to-day work in healthcare, which leaves little time to look for optimization potentials in processes and systems.

Medical data is inherently valuable. The price of a medical record on the dark web goes up to 50 US dollars, compared to 1 US dollar per credit card number. This increases the pressure on healthcare IT and pushes organizations towards the use of proven technology.

Most Blockchain projects are less than two years old and unproven in the working environment. As a young and innovative technology, Blockchain still has a small number of experts and developers, which cultivates the image of unstable and unsecured investment, in the eyes of the potential clients.

For a wide variety of reasons, many companies will wait for mainstream providers and business associates to develop the technology themselves, instead of taking a risk and switching to a new vendor.

Hype Overload

Business assessments made by individuals perceived as accomplished experts in their respective fields often go too far, describing the bright future of projects that are often unsecured and flawed. They act very freely since there are no repercussions for them. However, consequences for the decision makers can be terrifying.

The line between guessing and making valid conclusions must be strict, especially when new technologies are in question. Unsecure and unreliable projects are the biggest trap for investors and can inflict severe damage if they fail.

Most platforms have points or tokens today, and they tend to hype the technology to increase the value of the token. Today, personal experience of users highly motivated to compliment the quality of service can lead to deception of those eager to try it for the first time. The Blockchain is a strong example of this.

Conclusion

The most efficient way to achieve interoperability would be to establish an open standard technology infrastructure for IT systems in healthcare. Industry best practices suggest using open API (Application Programming Interface) to address the problem. However, an open API on its own is not enough. This is why Blockchain is used as a shared distributed infrastructure that allows a unified view of an individual's medical records across a lifetime in health IT systems.

Blockchain as a technology is great at addressing interoperability issues, is based on open standards, helps provide a bridge between institutions and is on its way to becoming widely accepted in many industries, including healthcare.

Use of the Blockchain in healthcare as described in this booklet has the potential to revolutionize the entire industry and bring many benefits with guaranteed privacy protection and top-notch security. Of course, there are still numerous obstacles on the way; however, the idea has its place in healthcare.

One of the first applications could be for decentralized medical record management. Many countries have already invested in some type of Blockchain application in healthcare – first among them is the small country of Estonia with intentions of bringing all its electronic patient files to the Blockchain. Many others should follow.

Blockchain has secured its place in health IT; all that remains now is to see if it works on a large scale. If just one country successfully implements Blockchain in its healthcare system, that would be a green light for the rest of the industry, and mass adoption might follow.

Further Reading

1. https://www.fbi.gov/investigate/white-collar-crime/health-care-fraud
2. https://www.healthit.gov/sites/default/files/1-78-blockchainandhealthitalgorithmsprivacydata_whitepaper.pdf
3. https://www.healthit.gov/sites/default/files/4-37-hhs_blockchain_challenge_deloitte_consulting_llp.pdf
4. http://catalyst.nejm.org/decoding-blockchain-technology-health/
5. http://www.intelligenthq.com/innovation-management/5-examples-of-using-blockchain-in-health-care/
6. https://www.finextra.com/blogposting/13801/blockchain-in-healthcare-make-the-industry-better
7. https://tierion.com/blog/blockchain-healthcare-2016-report/
8. https://medium.com/@Connected_Dots/blockchain-in-healthcare-for-dummies-190226e112eb
9. http://mcdonnell.mit.edu/blockchain_ehr.pdf
10. https://medium.com/mit-media-lab-digital-currency-initiative/medrec-electronic-medical-records-on-the-blockchain-c2d7e1bc7d09
11. https://www.media.mit.edu/projects/medrec/overview/
12. http://dci.mit.edu/assets/papers/eckblaw.pdf
13. https://www.wired.com/2017/02/moving-patient-data-messy-blockchain-help
14. https://news.bitcoin.com/gem-health-blockchain-medical-mgmt/
15. https://news.bitcoin.com/prescrypt-blockchain-prescriptions/

16. https://www.linkedin.com/pulse/blockchain-healthcare-your-banking-card-lucien-engelen

17. https://thenextweb.com/contributors/blockchain-technology-healthcare-dream-reality/

18. https://f1000researchdata.s3.amazonaws.com/manuscripts/8730/656d8fc5-932f-4f3a-8731-90215fa8de9d_8114_-_greg_irving.pdf?doi=10.12688/f1000research.8114.1

19. http://www.cccinnovationcenter.com/challenges/block-chain-challenge/view-winners/

If you've read this far…

… we are pretty sure that you now have an opinion on what we have written here. Please share it!

If you found this text helpful, we kindly ask that you leave a review on Amazon.com or the online book retailer of your choice. And more importantly: If you are **missing something** that we should cover here, if you find passages to be **less than clear**, or if you have **any other suggestions for improvement**, please don't hesitate to drop us an e-mail at **blockchain@intellicore.press**. We are looking forward to hearing from you!

Christina Czeschik and Ratko Stambolija | March 13, 2017

blockchain@intellicore.press

You may also like:

Cryptocurrencies for Fun and Profit

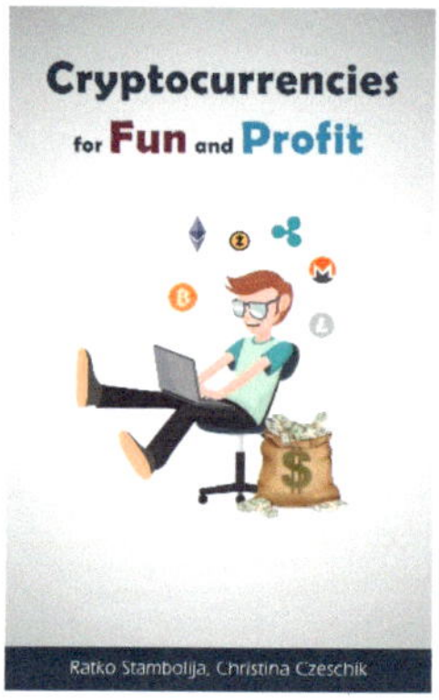

Intellicore Press, December 2017

ISBN 978-3962140083

Coming soon…

Please check Intellicore Press for updates!

Made in United States
Cleveland, OH
05 November 2026

47647253R00029